Respirat<

Emergencies

Respiratory Emergencies

E.H. Sawicka MD, MRCP
and
M.A. Branthwaite MD, FRCP, FFARCS

The Brompton Hospital
London, UK

Butterworths

London, Boston, Durban, Singapore, Sydney, Toronto, Wellington

in association with
Current Medical Literature Ltd
London

First published, 1987

© **1987 Current Medical Literature Ltd**

British Library Cataloguing in Publication Data

Sawicka, E. H.
  Respiratory emergencies.
  1. Respiratory insufficiency–Treatment
  2. Critical care medicine
  I. Title   II. Branthwaite, M. A.
  616.2'00425   RC776.R4

  ISBN 0-407-00861-6

Library of Congress Cataloging-in-Publication Data

Sawicka, E. H.
  Respiratory emergencies.

  Bibliography: p.
  Includes index.
  1. Respiratory organs–Diseases.   2. Medical emergencies.   I. Branthwaite, M. A. (Margaret Annie) II. Title.   [DNLM: 1. Emergencies.   2. Respiratory Tract Diseases–therapy.   WF 145 S271r]
  RC732.S29   1987   616.2'00425   87-24292
  ISBN 0-407-00861-6

Printed in Great Britain at the University Press, Cambridge

Contents

Preface

Preface

This book is directed primarily at those who need to provide immediate treatment for patients with respiratory illness. The greater part is based on the assumption that conventional hospital facilities will be available, but some emergencies which present outside hospital are also discussed. Conditions which are usually regarded as 'surgical' rather than 'medical' - for example, chest trauma - are excluded. No previous experience of the management of respiratory illness is assumed and, in general, only the initial decisions and treatment are discussed. In view of this inevitably didactic approach, alternative methods are not discussed, although the authors appreciate that some of the recommendations are controversial.

E.H. Sawicka
M.A. Branthwaite

1.Introduction

Respiratory insufficiency causes arterial hypoxaemia in any air-breathing subject, and this in turn interferes with cerebral, cardiac and renal function. Prompt recognition and treatment of the respiratory disorder are thus essential.

RESPIRATORY FAILURE

The strict definition of respiratory failure refers to the inability of an air-breathing subject to maintain normal arterial blood gas tensions, at sea level and in the absence of any cardiac or vascular anomaly which permits venous blood to enter the systemic arterial system directly. It is customary to distinguish arterial hypoxaemia with hypercapnia from arterial hypoxaemia with a normal or low arterial carbon dioxide tension, but the distinction is not absolute in that patients who start with hypocapnia may become hypercapnic with exhaustion or when respiratory insufficiency worsens, while those initially hypercapnic may become less so or even normocapnic if circulatory failure develops too.

Aetiology

Respiratory failure will result when there is 'interference with the desire to breathe or the ability to do so'. The desire to breathe refers to the generation of rhythmic inspiratory impulses in the brain stem, and the ability to breathe depends upon the presence of a patent airway, at least some alveoli which are both ventilated and perfused, an intact and mobile chest wall, and the appropriate peripheral neuromuscular responses to achieve respiratory movement. Some examples of disorders which can interfere with this system at one or more levels are listed in Table 1.1.

Any disorder that interferes with: The desire to breathe	
Causes	*Examples*
Damage to or depression of respiratory centre	Drugs, trauma, cerebrovascular accident

Any disorder that interferes with: The ability to breathe	
Causes	*Examples*
Respiratory obstruction at any level	Foreign body, asthma
An inadequate number of alveoli which are both ventilated and perfused	Pneumonia, pulmonary oedema or embolism
Mechanical interference with the thoracic cage	Trauma, deformity
Neuromuscular disease affecting the respiratory muscles	Myasthenia gravis, polyneuritis

Table 1.1 Some causes of respiratory failure

Diagnosis and assessment

Shortness of breath
This is the cardinal symptom but is a poor index of severity in patients acclimatized to respiratory disability or in those with a serious motor deficit or impaired consciousness.

Dyspnoea
Dyspnoea is recognized by an observer when the respiratory rate or pattern is inappropriate to activity, the accessory muscles are in use, or breathing is noisy (wheeze, stridor or the stertorous breathing of incomplete upper airway obstruction).

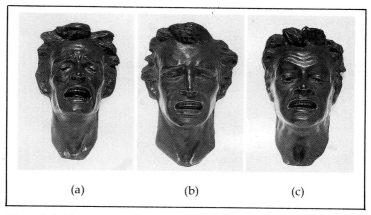

(a)　　　　　(b)　　　　　(c)

Figure 1.1 The progress of fatigue. Three bronze masks illustrating (a) breathlessness, (b) fatigue and (c) exhaustion, modelled by Dr R. Tait Mackenzie and reproduced with the kind permission of the curator of the Department of Anatomy, University of Cambridge.

Exhaustion

Exhaustion is suggested by loss of muscle tone, particularly in the face and neck, a sagging, open mouth, and a demoralized expression (Figure 1.1).

Dyspnoea with restlessness or confusion, often accompanied by sweating

This picture suggests serious hypoxaemia unless other causes such as pain and anxiety can be identified.

Cyanosis

Cyanosis is an unreliable indicator because it is difficult to detect in poor lighting, is apparent only when there is significant desaturation, is exaggerated by polycythaemia and hypercapnia, but is lessened by hypocapnia (which causes peripheral vasoconstriction and a left shift of the oxygen dissociation curve).

Hypertension, peripheral vasodilation, sweating and a coarse tremor

These are associated with hypercapnia but are often absent when respiratory failure is chronic.

Conjunctival injection
A better sign of chronic hypercapnia is conjunctival injection.

Papilloedema
Papilloedema is rare.

Acute right ventricular failure
Signs of acute right ventricular failure develop rapidly in patients with severe, unrelieved respiratory insufficiency. Accentuation of the pulmonary second sound, a fourth heart sound best heard just below the xiphisternum, and finally a third heart sound and rapid elevation of the jugular venous pressure may all appear in sequence over a matter of hours.

Some of these physical signs are modified by the presence of other pathology, and interpretation must allow for features such as mediastinal displacement, venous obstruction or a cardiac cause for respiratory disease.

Investigation

The following tests should be considered if facilities are available.

Radiology
A chest X-ray - preferably an upright postero-anterior view, possibly with a lateral too - is requested for hospitalized patients who do not have immediately life-threatening respiratory distress, or as soon as possible after urgent treatment has been implemented. An X-ray in the upright position should be sought if possible, even when a portable antero-posterior view is necessary. Some straightforward emergencies, e.g. severe acute asthma, which responds well to conventional treatment, can be managed without a film immediately after admission.

Spirometry
Measurements of vital capacity (VC), forced expired volume

in one second (FEV1) and peak expiratory flow rate (PEFR) are useful for documenting severity and progress in patients with airflow limitation (e.g. asthma or bronchitis). The peak flow manoeuvre is easier for an acutely breathless patient and less likely to cause coughing than trying to exhale a full vital capacity. A paediatric peak flow meter is necessary for patients with very severe airflow limitation because it records at values below 60 litres per minute. Direct correspondence between the upper figures on the paediatric meter and the lower figures on the adult meter should not be expected.

Patients with respiratory muscle weakness or isolated chest wall trauma are better monitored with serial measurements of vital capacity. The peak flow is a poor index of respiratory impairment in these circumstances.

Measurement of arterial blood gas tensions

This investigation is now accepted as routine in most patients with respiratory distress or insufficiency and the need for serial measurements may warrant the insertion of an arterial cannula. The results provide valuable information about severity and progress (Table 1.2) but specific values are virtually never the sole criterion for therapeutic decision-making.

Oxygen:	Normal arterial oxygen tension varies with age Values below 9.5 kPa (c. 70 mm Hg) while breathing air are abnormal but 'respiratory failure' usually refers to figures less than 8.0 kPa (60 mm Hg)
Carbon dioxide:	Normal arterial carbon dioxide tension lies between 5.0 and 6.3 kPa (c.38–46 mm Hg) 'Respiratory failure' is usually restricted to figures greater than 6.6 kPa (50 mm Hg)

Table 1.2 Interpretation of arterial blood gas tensions

The arterial oxygen tension (PaO_2) can be interpreted correctly only if the inspired oxygen concentration at the time of measurement is known, although the figure quoted for some oxygen delivery systems is only approximate. Care should be taken when interpreting values for pH and bicarbonate in the acutely ill. The chronic metabolic alkalosis associated with longstanding hypercapnia is inapparent if there is a coincident metabolic acidosis caused by severe hypoxaemia or circulatory insufficiency. When recovery follows, the metabolic acidosis is likely to resolve within a matter of hours, thus revealing the underlying metabolic alkalosis. The apparent absence of a metabolic component initially can hinder recognition of both the

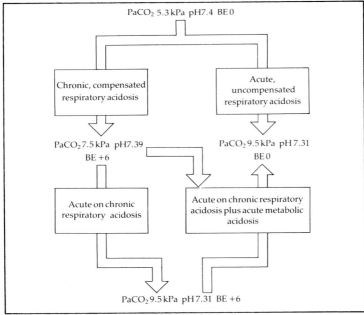

Figure 1.2 Some biochemical consequences of respiratory failure. The changes in arterial carbon dioxide tension ($PaCO_2$), pH and base excess (BE) which occur when carbon dioxide is retained acutely or more slowly, and the effect on these variables of subsequent acute deterioration in respiratory function or the development of a metabolic acidosis.

chronicity of hypercapnia and the severity of the acute episode (Figure 1.2).

Other tests
An *ECG* will often help to differentiate cardiac causes of respiratory distress but electrocardiographic evidence is sometimes short-lived, e.g. after pulmonary embolism. Transitory ECG evidence of right axis deviation and right ventricular strain can also be seen with severe respiratory distress, e.g. asthma (Figure 1.3). An immediate *full blood count and differential white cell count* and *microscopy of sputum* should be requested if infection is suspected. Cultures of sputum, throat swab and sometimes blood should be arranged, and blood should be collected for subsequent immunodiagnostic tests. Additional investigations will be necessary in some circumstances.

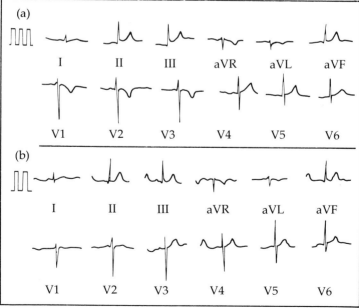

Figure 1.3 ECG changes in severe acute asthma : (a) during the attack; (b) after recovery.

2. Central Respiratory Depression/Loss of Respiratory Drive

These terms are used synonymously to describe patients in whom there is an inappropriate reduction in the frequency or depth of breathing as a result of interference with brain-stem function. Drug overdosage is still the most common cause although numbers have fallen in the UK as barbiturate narcotics have been withdrawn. Drug combinations, or the simultaneous consumption of alcohol, account for a proportion of cases.

Other causes include head injury, cerebrovascular accidents, and cerebral depression after any cardiorespiratory crisis such as cardiac arrest, drowning or exposure to toxic fumes. Extreme hypothermia causes respiratory depression but the simultaneous depression of metabolic rate means that oxygenation and carbon dioxide clearance are often appropriate.

Clinical features

Rate, rhythm and depth of respiration are all likely to be abnormal, and the simultaneous impairment of consciousness means that upper airway obstruction is often present too, either because the relaxed tongue falls back to block the pharynx, or because blood, secretions or vomit have been inhaled.

Management

Immediate intervention may be necessary either to restore patency of the airway or to institute artificial ventilation if the patient is already apnoeic. Unless prohibited by the presence of injuries, particularly an unstable cervical spine, the patient who is still breathing, albeit shallowly, should be turned into the 'tonsil' position to help maintain patency of the airway (Figure 2.1).

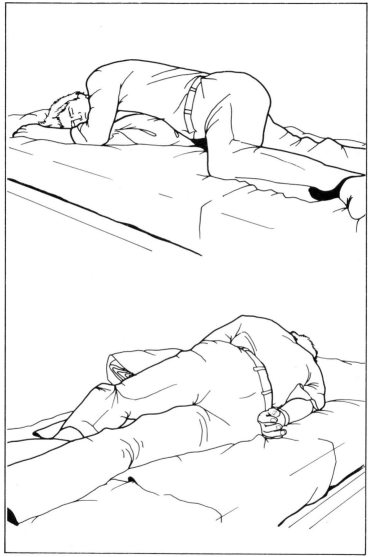

Figure 2.1 The 'tonsil' position. The patient lies semi-prone with the lower arm posteriorly and a pillow anteriorly. The upper leg is flexed at the knee so that the posture is retained.

Endotracheal intubation and mechanical ventilation are often needed but, before these more invasive forms of treatment are implemented, consideration should be given to the following:

1. Is recovery likely and, if so, what is the probable duration of respiratory depression? For example, assisted ventilation is rarely appropriate for an elderly subject with respiratory depression after spontaneous cerebral haemorrhage.

2. Is there evidence of either pre-existing pulmonary disease or any acute pulmonary injury? Either may enhance the need for ventilatory assistance.

3. Is there a role for a specific antidote such as naloxone after poisoning with opiate or related drugs?

4. Is there other pathology (e.g. visceral or skeletal trauma) which will influence management in the immediate or longer-term? The need for urgent diagnostic radiology, surgery, or management of skeletal injuries with traction favours intubation.

5. What facilities and expertise are available to secure safe, atraumatic intubation and appropriate assisted ventilation?

In general, patients suffering from drug-induced respiratory depression should be intubated and ventilated rather than given non-specific respiratory stimulants. Those known to be depressed by opiates often respond to intravenous naloxone (0.4–2.0 mg, repeated at intervals of 2–3 minutes to a total of 10 mg). The effect is transitory, often far shorter than the depressant drug. Close observation is required and further doses or an infusion of naloxone given if necessary; alternatively, intubation and assisted ventilation may be preferred.

Patients with severe central respiratory depression are

often so flaccid that intubation is easy. This is not always the case and, unless the airway cannot be secured by an alternative means, intubation should be delayed until suction is available and the appropriate apparatus has been selected and checked.

Oral endotracheal intubation is preferred to the nasal route in an emergency because it is quicker and easier. The oral tube can be exchanged later for a nasal one, as an elective procedure and under controlled conditions, if thought necessary.

Subjects suffering from uncomplicated central respiratory depression can be ventilated with air, but oxygen enrichment is desirable if there has been any pulmonary damage or soiling, or if the circulation is falling too. A tidal volume of 8–10 ml kg^{-1}, delivered at a rate of 12–15 breaths per minute, is appropriate for an adult of average build. These figures are approximate only, do not require more than an estimate of body weight, and may need to be modified if there is coincident pulmonary pathology or an abnormal metabolic rate.

3. Acute Upper Airway Obstruction

Adequate ventilation can be maintained through the adult airway until its diameter has been grossly reduced. Tracheal narrowing to a diameter of 3 mm or less is to be expected by the time dyspnoea is present at rest.

COMPLETE OBSTRUCTION

Sudden, complete obstruction of the upper airway results most commonly from the aspiration of solid food – while eating too fast, talking while eating, or eating when partially obtunded by alcohol. The term 'café coronary' refers to sudden death, usually from acute obstruction rather than from any primary cardiac lesion. Other causes of upper airway obstruction in adults include trauma to the face, tongue and jaw, sudden massive swelling of mouth, tongue or larynx as part of an anaphylactic response, glottic oedema (or occasionally spasm) secondary to pharyngeal or mediastinal infection, or rapid enlargement of a tumour caused either by haemorrhage or by oedema, the latter sometimes provoked by treatment. Acute upper airway obstruction can also occur in any unconscious subject, especially if there are loose teeth, dentures, blood, vomit, mud or water in the mouth.

Clinical features

The cardinal symptoms in conscious subjects are extreme dyspnoea and fear. Inspiratory stridor is audible if the obstruction is incomplete but total obstruction is silent. Characteristically, the patient clutches the throat, gasping and sometimes attempting to cough. Loss of consciousness follows rapidly if complete obstruction is unrelieved, and cardiac arrest will then occur within minutes, even in the previously healthy.

13

Management

Acute, total obstruction of the upper airway is an emergency which is met most often outside hospital. Management depends on whether the subject is still conscious or whether death is imminent.

Conscious patient

If the subject is conscious and inhalation of a foreign body is suspected, deliver a few sharp blows on the back, between the scapulae. Occasionally this is sufficient to dislodge the obstruction.

A more effective but potentially more dangerous manoeuvre is that described by Heimlich. The subject leans forward and the operator encircles the patient's body with his arms below those of the patient (Figure 3.1). Clasping his hands together and holding them firmly in the subject's epigastrium, the operator delivers three or four sharp thrusts in an upwards and backwards direction. This is intended to create pressure below the obstruction and force it out of the glottis. Carried out too vigorously or with the force applied inappropriately, rupture of the liver or damage to stomach or sternum can occur.

Unconscious patient

Subjects who are already unconscious should be placed semi-prone. The operator should sweep his fingers round the back of the subject's mouth to dislodge dentures, food or foreign material impacted there. This done, the jaw is pulled forward and upward to ensure that the tongue is not contributing to the obstruction. If the subject remains unconscious and apnoeic, an attempt is made to inflate the chest using either expired air or a manual resuscitator if available.

No time should be wasted persisting with these efforts if they are not successful immediately. If it is clear that the airway remains obstructed, that cardiac arrest is about to occur or has already done so, and that laryngoscopy and intubation are either impossible or not available, an attempt

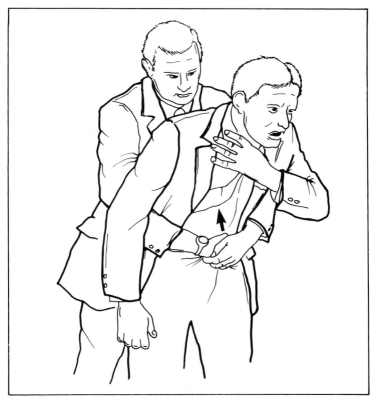

Figure 3.1 The Heimlich manoeuvre.

should be made to secure air entry through the cricothyroid membrane. The equipment chosen will be governed by what is to hand - a large-bore intravenous cannula is the least traumatic but may secure an airway just sufficient to support life. A penknife followed by the pointed shaft of a ball-point pen without its cartridge has been used successfully. If the equipment is available, a mini-tracheotomy is an easier, safer and therefore preferable alternative for the inexperienced than attempts at conventional tracheostomy. The technique of insertion is illustrated in Figure 3.2 and the equipment is shown in detail in Figure 3.3.

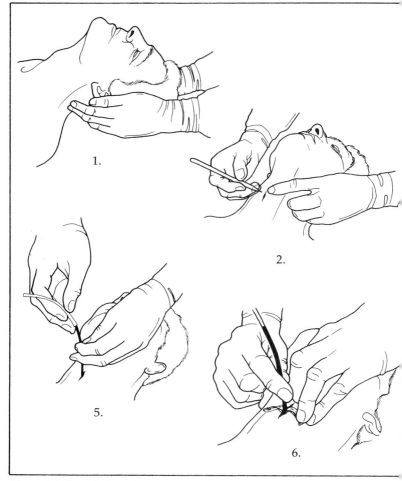

Figure 3.2 Steps in inserting a Mini-trach:
1. The patient is positioned supine with head, neck and chin extended. The operator stands above the head, facing the patient's feet.
2. The cricothyroid membrane is palpated and the point of insertion marked.
3. A midline vertical stab incision is made into the airway through the cricothyroid membrane using the guarded scalpel, cutting edge towards the feet. The blade is too short to injure the posterior wall of the trachea.
4. The introducer is passed into the trachea.

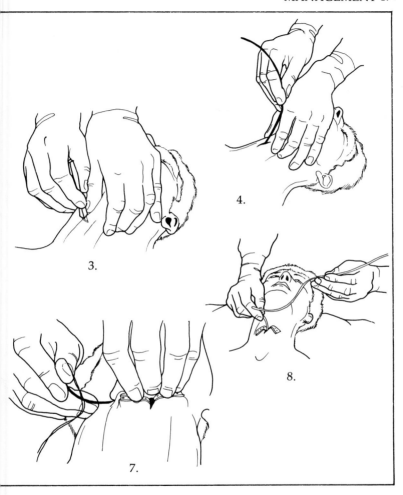

5. *The wings of the cannula are bent laterally as the cannula is passed over the introducer into the trachea.*

6. *The cannula is held in place and the introducer is withdrawn.*

7. *The cannula is fixed in position by suturing the wings to the skin.*

8. *The suction catheter is passed immediately to clear any existing blood and secretions. A mucus extractor (as used for neonatal resuscitation) can be used for suction if the conventional apparatus is not available.*
(Reproduced by kind permission of Portex Ltd, Hythe, Kent.)

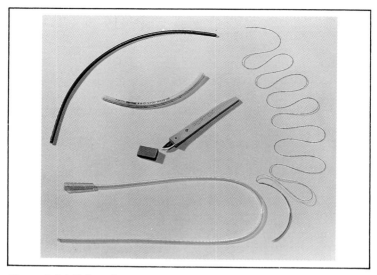

Figure 3.3 Mini-trach apparatus. (Reproduced by kind permission of Portex Ltd, Hythe, Kent.)

If possible, oxygen rather than air should be delivered through the narrow airway created by any of these methods. Care must also be taken to allow gas to escape from the lungs, which it can do only through the same narrow route.

It is important to remember that high drama breeds over-hasty action. The front of the neck of a patient with acute respiratory obstruction is engorged with blood which can all too easily enter the airway and compound the problem. It is also quite difficult to penetrate the skin of the anterior neck in the average adult, especially with 'instruments' which are neither sharp nor designed for the purpose. It is essential therefore that those dealing with this emergency should keep a particularly cool head and indulge in heroic assaults on the trachea only if death is otherwise inevitable.

Measures of value in *specific circumstances* include:

1. Subcutaneous adrenaline (0.5 mg) in cases of *anaphylaxis*. Adrenaline can be given intravenously but this should be

avoided unless monitoring facilities and resuscitation equipment are fairly readily available.

2. Nasopharyngeal intubation. Of particular value in patients with grossly distorted oropharyngeal anatomy *following trauma*. A small-diameter, uncuffed, nasal endotracheal tube or a naspharyngeal airway should be chosen and introduced *gently* through the nostril. The largest passage is often the one beyond what appears externally to be the smaller naris. Sometimes passage of the tube into the pharynx is sufficient to relieve obstruction caused by a swollen tongue, but this provides no protection against aspiration of pharyngeal contents into the lungs. However, 'blind' nasal intubation – guiding a nasotracheal tube through the larynx without a laryngoscope – is not always easy, even for the experienced, and efforts to do so can cause profuse nasal bleeding, especially if a cuffed tube is used.

SEVERE, INCOMPLETE OBSTRUCTION, INCLUDING LESIONS OF THE LOWER TRACHEA

An inhaled foreign body which does not impact in the glottis is likely to pass through the trachea and enter the bronchial tree. Depending on the site of impaction, such patients will present with cough, moderate dyspnoea, possibly haemoptysis or, later, infection. Stricture, malignant disease and severe thoracic trauma are the most common causes of tracheal obstruction below the glottis, and the patient is more likely to present subacutely. The most urgent cases are those in which there is a fairly sudden increase in the severity of the obstruction, e.g. after venous thrombosis, haemorrhage or oedema. Although this means that urgent intervention may well be required, the obstruction is likely to be fairly soft and therefore relatively easy to pass, unlike the much more slowly progressive but hard nature of, for example, a tracheal stricture or scirrhous carcinoma.

Clinical features

Dyspnoea, stridor and anxiety are characteristic. Signs which suggest that the obstruction is becoming intolerable are orthopnoea, reluctance to try to drink, a rising tachycardia or tachypnoea and, ultimately, restlessness and confusion.

Management

Definitive management should be undertaken in hospital by those equipped to handle not only the airway but also the pathology responsible for the obstruction. Symptomatic relief can be provided by:

1. Use of a helium/oxygen mixture: this is much less dense than air and so facilitates gas movement under conditions of turbulent flow.

2. Intravenous corticosteroids, e.g. hydrocortisone (200 mg 6-hourly) or dexamethasone (4 mg 6-hourly) to decrease local oedema.

3. Posture: support the patient upright in a position of comfort, usually leaning forward with the arms resting on a table.

4. Conveying confidence and reassurance.

The need to allay anxiety is twofold: in part it is to provide relief, but the less anxious patient will also breathe more quietly and slowly so that the rate of gas flow past the obstruction will fall, less effort will be needed and the sensation of obstruction will diminish. A considered decision is needed about the magnitude of and justification for the risks of sedation using small doses of an anxiolytic given intravenously. Benzodiazepines are less likely than opiates to depress respiration or impair the cough reflex, but the effects are less easily reversed.

   If urgent relief of the obstruction has to be undertaken,

every effort should be made to identify the location of the lesion before attempting to bypass it. A selection of small-diameter but long endotracheal tubes should be available, and gum elastic bougies can be helpful because they are available in small size, have some degree of stiffness but are also malleable. A fibre-optic laryngoscope or bronchoscope is invaluable but rarely available. Suction, a good light, a reliable laryngoscope, resuscitation equipment and an assistant should be sought if possible.

Intubation should be carried out through the mouth or nose under local anaesthesia. If the patient is so restless that this is impractical, it may be possible to induce light general anaesthesia using an inhalation technique. An intravenous induction agent followed by a muscle relaxant is *most hazardous* and should only be considered by an experienced operator who has already satisfied himself that the airway can be maintained and that effective passive ventilation can be achieved with a facemask.

4.Severe Acute Asthma

A few patients with unstable asthma develop a severe attack with overwhelming speed and die before medical assistance is available. More commonly deterioration occurs over a matter of days or even weeks.

Clinical features

Dyspnoea at rest, audible wheezing and cyanosis are usual. The chest is visibly over-distended, the accessory muscles are in use, but, as the condition worsens, effort and the noise of breathing diminish. Symptomatic improvement is not always matched by objective evidence of change and so progress should be monitored by serial measurement of heart rate, respiratory rate, degree of paradox in the arterial blood pressure, and peak expiratory flow rate (Figure 4.1). Determination of arterial blood gas tensions should be considered in patients giving rise to concern, the usual findings being arterial hypoxaemia and hypocapnia. Hypercapnia does occur, particularly in children, but is not an absolute indication for mechanical assistance to ventilation. Of much greater concern is an arterial carbon dioxide tension rising into or above the normal range, a finding often associated with exhaustion. Criteria of particularly severe asthma are given in Table 4.1, those associated with an especially adverse prognosis being indicated by an asterisk.

Management

Immediate management before transfer to hospital
Reassurance, the administration of oxygen, a beta-adrenergic agonist and the initiation of a course of corticosteroids should all be considered. Immediate referral

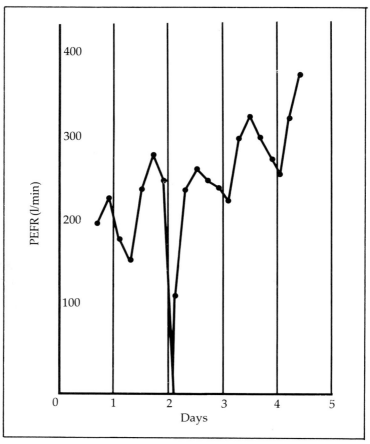

Figure 4.1 Serial measurements of peak expiratory flow rate (PEFR) in a hospitalized subject, showing marked diurnal variation. Cardiac arrest occurred at 02.00 hours on day three.

to hospital is necessary for patients with an unusually severe or intransigent attack. Oxygen should be given during transport and treatment with corticosteroids (hydrocortisone 4 mg kg^{-1} intravenously) initiated before transfer. A beta-adrenergic agonist such as salbutamol (5 mg) delivered from solution by a portable nebulizer, preferably driven by oxygen, will often provide relief, even

* Disturbance of consciousness

   Central cyanosis

   Arterial oxygen tension less than 8.0 kPa

* Any elevation of arterial carbon dioxide tension

   Gross overinflation on chest X-ray

   Pulsus paradoxus

   ECG abnormalities

* Pneumothorax or pneumomediastinum

* Obvious exhaustion

* FEV_1 less than 0.5 litre } no significant increase
* FVC less than 1.0 litre   } with bronchodilator

---

* Signifies dangerous feature.
From Rebuck and Read (1971).

Table 4.1   Criteria of severe or dangerous asthma

---

when the patient reports that use of a pressurized aerosol is no longer effective. Parenteral sympathomimetics, certainly by the intravenous route, are probably better reserved for use in hospital, and intravenous aminophylline should be avoided unless it is certain that the patient has not been using a theophylline derivative in the recent past.

Subcutaneous adrenaline (0.5 mg) should be considered for patients *in extremis* if artificial ventilation is not available.

Management on admission to hospital

Patients with an attack of asthma sufficiently severe to warrant referral to hospital should be admitted. Initial assessment includes the measurements outlined above. In addition, blood should be taken for an immediate estimation of plasma theophylline level in those using the drug regularly or treated with it within the preceding 24 hours. A chest X-ray is desirable, and investigation to identify a respiratory infection may be appropriate, although purulent sputum can be caused by eosinophils as readily as by neutrophils.

1. Oxygen

Oxygen should be continued in a concentration of 35–60%, there being negligible risk of inducing hypercapnia.

2. Steroid therapy

Treatment with corticosteroid should be continued or initiated. A loading dose of $4 \, mg \, kg^{-1}$ hydrocortisone given intravenously is followed by $3 \, mg \, kg^{-1}$ every 6 hours, aiming to achieve a blood level of about $100 \, \mu g \, dl^{-1}$. A course of oral steroids is commenced at the same time, e.g. $0.5 \, mg \, kg^{-1}$ prednisolone per day.

3. Salbutamol

A beta-adrenergic agonist should be given, either intravenously (e.g. salbutamol $250 \, \mu g$ as a bolus injected slowly, or $5–10 \, \mu g \, min^{-1}$ as an infusion) or by inhalation. Although there is still some controversy about which route is preferable, it appears that the duration of action of a single dose is longer and the incidence of side-effects lower with the inhaled route. The pressurized aerosol delivers a relatively small dose ($100 \, \mu g$/puff) and penetration within the bronchial tree will be impaired if the tidal volume is small or the technique of use poor. A dose of 2.5 or 5 mg of salbutamol nebulized from solution with an oxygen-enriched mixture not only permits a larger quantity to enter the lungs but also achieves better distribution. 5 mg (1 ml of the 0.5% respirator solution) should be diluted to at least 3 ml with normal saline and nebulized with a flow rate of preferably 8–10 l min-1. Delivery of a nebulized bronchodilator with intermittent positive pressure breathing achieves little if any additional benefit but, if a gas-driven nebulizer is not available, use of a pressurized aerosol with a pear-shaped spacer achieves comparable drug deposition.

4. Atropine

Patients who fail to respond to the first dose of salbutamol delivered by inhalation should be given a further dose of 5 mg after half an hour. At the same time, atropine sulphate 3 mg (0.3 ml of the 1% preparation) should be added to the solution in the nebulizer. Patients with severe acute asthma often achieve significant additional bronchodilatation if atropine (or a derivative such as *ipratropium bromide*) is added to the beta-adrenergic agonist, and there is no evidence that its use increases sputum viscosity or the incidence of tachycardia.

5. *Aminophylline*
If symptom relief is still inadequate and there has been no improvement in the peak flow rate, consideration should be given to the use of *aminophylline*. Although effective, the therapeutic range is narrow ($10–20 \mu g\, ml^{-1}$). The incidence of serious and sometimes fatal cerebral or cardiovascular side-effects has risen with the widespread use of long-acting oral theophylline derivatives, and it is preferable to withhold aminophylline from patients regularly using such a preparation until a blood level has been obtained. Those not using regular theophyllines can be given a loading dose of $5–6\, mg\, kg^{-1}$ by *slow* intravenous injection, followed by an infusion of $0.5\, mg\, kg^{-1} h^{-1}$. An infusion at a similar rate, but without the loading dose, can be given to those previously treated with theophyllines, provided the plasma concentration of the drug does not exceed the therapeutic range at the outset. Once a theophylline infusion has been established, it is desirable to check after approximately 4 and 12 hours that the drug concentration lies within the therapeutic range. Lower doses may be needed in the elderly or in patients with impaired cardiac or hepatic function.

6. *Rehydration*
A proportion of asthmatic patients are dehydrated on admission because they have been too breathless to drink and insensible loss has been increased by restlessness. Rehydration will help to prevent inspissation of bronchial secretions and can be achieved safely while intravenous medication is being used. Antibiotics are often prescribed but there is little evidence that infection is responsible for more than a small proportion of episodes. Potassium supplements should be given if hypokalaemia follows

treatment with beta-adrenergic agonists, and measures to control hyperglycaemia and glycosuria caused by stress, steroids and beta-adrenergic agonists are sometimes necessary.

7. Sedatives
Sedative drugs are contraindicated – restlessness and anxiety indicate hypoxaemia, and persistence of these features after reassurance and treatment with the measures outlined here indicates asthma of unusual severity, possibly requiring mechanical ventilation.

Measures for the patient who fails to respond
The pathology of acute asthma consists of spasm of smooth muscle, mucosal oedema and obstruction of small airways by inspissated mucus. If medication given to relieve the spasm and oedema fails to provide relief, it can be assumed that *mucous plugging* is a major factor contributing to the obstruction.

1. Increasing the humidity
Increasing the humidity of the inspired gas is sometimes effective in liquefying secretions and promoting their expectoration. This is particularly helpful for patients with asthma associated with bronchopulmonary aspergillosis. Humidifiers generating a cold mist should not be used in case cold-induced bronchoconstriction results.

2. Lavage
More aggressive measures for the removal of bronchial secretions include segmental lavage through a fibre-optic bronchoscope or the regular instillation of normal saline into the bronchial tree during mechanical ventilation. The latter should be reserved for patients in whom mechanical assistance to breathing is considered essential in its own right.

3. Mechanical ventilation
Criteria for initiating artificial ventilation are not easy to

define. Cardiorespiratory collapse will precipitate the need in a few patients. Resuscitation is sometimes very easy in this group and prolonged support is unnecessary; in a small proportion, ventilation is virtually impossible, even when manual assistance is attempted after endotracheal intubation.

More often, mechanical ventilation is required because the patient is becoming exhausted by the effort of breathing. Hypoxaemia worsens, restlessness exacerbates the oxygen lack, and the arterial carbon dioxide tension starts to climb. The decision to intervene is usually based on the clinical appearance of 'exhaustion' rather than on any specific measurement, but features which may be noticed at the same time include a heart rate which is continuing to climb, a diminution in the degree of paradox in the systemic arterial pressure, and a rising respiratory rate (Figure 4.2).

Pneumothorax and acute circulatory failure are complications of mechanical ventilation for severe acute asthma and both are more likely to occur if there is further distension of the lungs (Figure 4.3). The minute volume which can be delivered safely (i.e. so that further increase in lung volume does not occur) is often inadequate to achieve normocapnia. This should be accepted initially while measures such as the regular instillation of normal saline through the endotracheal tube (2 ml every 15 minutes for adult patients) are instituted to loosen bronchial secretions and aid their removal. Heavy sedation and possibly muscle paralysis too will be needed to avoid coughing, and the pattern of ventilation should allow time for effective distribution of gas during inspiration (duration of inspiration and expiration should be approximately equal). Use of positive end-expiratory pressure has been advocated on an anecdotal basis but there are many theoretical objections to its use and it should probably be avoided until clear evidence of benefit is available.

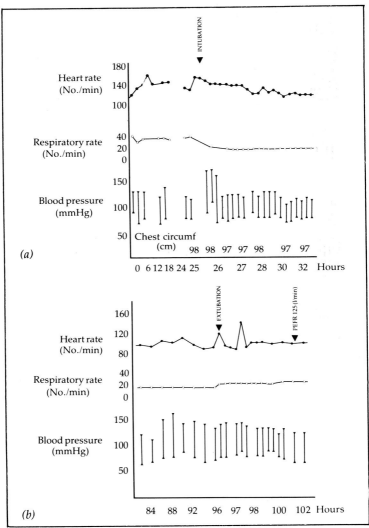

Figure 4.2 Severe acute asthma requiring mechanical ventilation. Tachypnoea and a rising heart rate over the first 24 hours (a) precede intubation and mechanical ventilation. Drug treatment was continued unaltered but saline was instilled regularly through the endotracheal tube. Gradual resolution culminated in uneventful extubation after 3 days (b). Note the changes in time scale.

Figure 4.3 Some hazards of severe
acute asthma.(a) Gross over-inflation
of the lungs in a patient who required
mechanical ventilation.
(b) Pneumomediastinum and
surgical emphysema occurring
spontaneously during an attack of
asthma.

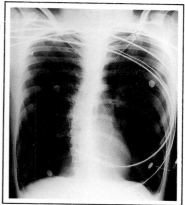

(a)

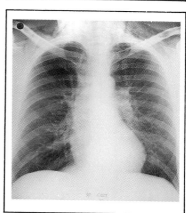

(b)

5. Acute on Chronic Respiratory Failure

Chronic airflow limitation (chronic airways obstruction) is the usual cause of hypercapnic respiratory failure. Prolonged hypoxaemia results in polycythaemia, and renal retention of bicarbonate compensates for the respiratory acidosis so that the pH is within the normal range. This stable equilibrium can be disturbed very easily, for example by an acute infective exacerbation of bronchitis, other respiratory infections such as influenza or pneumonia, intra-abdominal pathology or surgery, respiratory depressant drugs (e.g. analgesics or hypnotics) or an excess of alcohol. As a result, hypoxaemia worsens, the arterial carbon dioxide tension rises, and the pH falls.

Relief of hypoxaemia decreases respiratory drive further and so the carbon dioxide tension rises even higher, resulting in narcosis and respiratory depression. Fluid retention is common, and the degree of hypoxaemia and circulatory failure may be such that diuretics are ineffective, or cause fluid loss from the vascular compartment while the patient remains oedematous. Congestion and oedema occur in the pulmonary as well as the systemic vascular bed and this in turn worsens pulmonary function and exacerbates the airways obstruction. In some patients the arterial carbon dioxide tension falls a little at this stage, perhaps because respiration is stimulated either by pulmonary engorgement or tissue hypoxia.

Clinical features

Worsening breathlessness and cyanosis are typical. The full bounding pulse and facial flushing associated with acute hypercapnia are rare but conjunctival injection and a coarse tremor are common, as are disturbances of intellect and consciousness. Depression, belligerence and finally narcosis are characteristic of hypercapnia; restlessness and confusion are more suggestive of hypoxaemia.

It is customary to diagnose 'cor pulmonale' when pulmonary disease is associated with elevation of the jugular venous pressure, peripheral oedema, hepatomegaly, and rales in the lung fields. These physical signs can, however, have an alternative origin - elevation of the venous pressure, especially in expiration, reflecting intrathoracic pressure, displacement of the liver as a result of chronic over-distension of the lungs, rales representing the presence of bronchial mucus rather than pulmonary oedema, and peripheral oedema reflecting an increase in total body water or its inappropriate distribution as a consequence of hypercapnia. Features which suggest that cardiac failure is making a significant contribution to the clinical condition are nausea and anorexia (hepatic congestion), a poor peripheral circulation, elevation of the jugular venous pressure throughout the respiratory cycle, gross peripheral oedema, tenderness as well as enlargement of the liver, and diuretic-resistant oliguria with a rising blood urea level. The heart sound may be difficult to hear because the lungs are over-expanded and noisy but a fourth heart sound is very common and a third sound more likely when the circulation is beginning to fall. Both are best heard below or a little to the left of the xiphisternum.

Management

The cause of deterioration should be sought and any obvious factor (e.g. sedation) should be stopped. The patient should be sat up and, if responsive, encouraged to take a few deep breaths and cough. Any sputum expectorated as a result should be sent for microscopy and culture.

Oxygen
Oxygen should be given with caution and in controlled concentration, usually 24% or 28%. The arterial blood gas tensions should be monitored at the outset if possible to confirm that unacceptable hypercapnia does not occur. If

this is impractical, the patient should be watched closely for signs of increasingly shallow respiration and worsening narcosis. Masks supplying a known percentage of oxygen are preferred but some patients are more tolerant of nasal cannulae. A flow rate of 2 litres per minute through nasal cannulae achieves an inspired concentration of about 25%; a flow as low as 1 litre per minute may be needed to avoid hypercapnia in patients with very shallow respiration. Humidification of the added oxygen delivered by these means is not required routinely, but may be helpful for selected patients with tenacious secretions.

Bronchodilators

Bronchodilator drugs are an essential part of management. Salbutamol, atropine or theophyllines can all be considered and administered as described on page 26. Corticosteroid treatment is indicated if airflow limitation is a prominent feature, and may achieve worthwhile bronchodilatation during acute episodes, even in patients who fail to respond to steroids when assessed while stable and free from infection. Fluid retention is particularly likely when corticosteroids are used in these circumstances, and a diuretic may be needed.

Antibiotics

Antibiotics are essential if an acute infection or infective exacerbation of bronchitis is responsible for deterioration. *Haemophilus influenzae* and *Streptococcus pneumoniae* are the organisms associated most commonly with infective exacerbations of bronchitis. Amoxycillin, co-trimoxazole, tetracycline or erythromycin are likely to prove effective and one or other of these agents should be started as soon as possible, but preferably not before sputum has been collected for culture. The choice should take account of recent antibiotic treatment and any history of drug intolerance. Selecting an antibiotic before the results of culture are available is less easy if a viral infection or pneumonic illness is suspected and the discussion on page 43 will apply. One final difficulty is that culture of macroscopically purulent sputum does not always demonstrate a pathogen. Sometimes this is because antibiotic therapy has already been started, or alternatively the organism is fastidious and the culture conditions have inhibited its growth. Although it is desirable to withhold antibiotics until a specific organism has been identified, especially if there has been an inadequate response to one antibiotic already, this policy cannot always be upheld and an intelligent guess about the likely nature of the pathogen must govern the selection of treatment. Chloramphenicol has a wide spectrum of activity and is often effective when other agents have failed, although its potential for serious adverse effects on the bone marrow must be remembered, especially in those with chronic illness.

Sputum clearance

Sputum clearance is inefficient in patients with chronic bronchitis, emphysema or bronchiectasis. Recovery from acute infection is as much dependent upon the clearance of infected secretions as it is on the use of antibiotics and so this aspect of treatment requires equal attention. An experienced physiotherapist can often posture the patient and help him to cough effectively, although over-enthusiastic treatment should be avoided because of the increased oxygen demand, exhaustion, or even circulatory collapse which can follow. Increasing the humidity of the inspired gas loosens secretions, and delivery of bronchodilator drugs or nebulized normal saline by intermittent positive pressure breathing using a mask or mouthpiece is a useful adjunct, especially for patients acclimatized to this treatment. Nasopharyngeal or even nasotracheal suction is helpful if weakness prevents effective coughing, but great gentleness is needed to avoid distress or mucosal trauma.

More invasive forms of sputum removal such as bronchoscopy should be avoided because the procedure will worsen hypoxaemia and the operator has little or no control of the airway. If conservative measures such as those outlined above are ineffective, consideration should be given to the use of respiratory stimulants or, more importantly, endotracheal intubation and controlled ventilation (see below).

Diuretics

Diuretics are most useful in patients with florid fluid retention, especially if there is pulmonary venous engorgement too. Even if there is no evidence of pulmonary congestion, lowering the right atrial pressure will help to relieve passive congestion in bronchial veins and lymphatics and this in turn will lessen airway obstruction. However, over-enthusiastic use of diuretics results in hypovolaemia and a rising blood urea level, and can actually worsen circulatory failure if there is severe pulmonary arterial hypertension and impaired right ventricular function. Persistent elevation of the jugular venous pressure when there is little or no peripheral oedema and the blood urea is rising reflects either the high intra-thoracic pressure or, more likely, the venoconstriction which accompanies circulatory failure.

Respiratory stimulants

Respiratory stimulants such of doxapram (0.5–4 mg min^{-1}) or, more recently, the specific respiratory stimulant almitrine have only a limited place in the management of acute on chronic respiratory failure. They should be considered if facilities for controlled ventilation either do not exist or are considered inappropriate for the individual case. Treatment with a respiratory stimulant is most likely to be effective if some potentially reversible and transitory factor is operating, such as respiratory depression after uncontrolled oxygen therapy or unwise sedation. Sometimes respiratory stimulants will help to maintain adequate ventilation while antibiotics and attempts to drain secretions take effect, but more often stimulants in these circumstances merely increase the patient's distress because he is conscious of enhanced respiratory drive but either cannot respond to it or feels exhausted by the additional effort.

Mechanical ventilation

Intubation and mechanical ventilation should be considered for patients with potentially reversible disease who are *in extremis* when first seen or who deteriorate in spite of treatment. Features which suggest that intervention is necessary include deteriorating consciousness and/or increasing restlessness, signs of circulatory failure, or diuretic-resistant oliguria in the absence of dehydration. Once established on mechanical ventilation, sputum can be removed by suction and the hazard of depressing respiration with oxygen is removed so that hypoxaemia can be relieved completely by increasing the inspired concentration. This alone is often sufficient to restore urine output and a satisfactory peripheral circulation. Chronic hypercapnia should not be reversed rapidly because cerebral vasoconstriction, myocardial depression and an unacceptably high pH are likely to follow. Mechanical ventilation is extremely effective in the short term but it is sometimes difficult to restore spontaneous ventilation because of the severity of underlying lung damage, and the incidence of complications such as further infection, pneumothorax or gastrointestinal ulceration is high. Results are best in patients with bronchitis rather than emphysema, whose previous exercise tolerance permitted at least some outdoor activity and who are admitted with some unequivocal and reversible cause of acute deterioration rather than a minor exacerbation of sputum production or breathlessness.

Patients known to be housebound by chronic pulmonary disease should probably not be subjected to the indignity and discomfort of mechanical ventilation. Restlessness and anxiety, suggesting worsening hypoxaemia and/or circulatory failure, may warrant the cautious use of small amounts of a sedative - drugs which are otherwise totally contraindicated in the management of acute on chronic respiratory failure.

6.Pneumonia and Pulmonary Collapse

PNEUMONIA

Pneumonia in the previously healthy is often easy to diagnose and to treat, hence the term 'emergency' hardly applies. The same is not true for patients predisposed to infection or who are ill-equipped to respond to it for reasons such as those given in Tables 6.1 and 6.2. A very small proportion of previously healthy subjects develop overwhelming pneumonia but show none of these characteristics, and then it must be postulated that the organism is of unusual virulence or the infecting dose massive.

1. Non-specific	Age
	Malnutrition
	Alcohol
	Acute/chronic systemic illness
2. Specific	Congenital
	Acquired: disease
	side-effect of treatment

Table 6.1 Some causes of enhanced susceptibility to infection

Clinical features

Malaise, fever, chest pain, breathlessness and cough are the usual symptoms. The cough is often unproductive, at least initially; rust-coloured sputum is characteristic of a haemorrhagic exudate but is rarely seen.

Disruption of surface barrier	Oral flora
	Gastrointestinal tract flora
	Candida
Granulocyte defects	Gram-negative rods
	Pseudomonas
	Oral flora
	Aspergillus
Hypogammaglobulinaemia	*Pneumococcus*
	Haemophilus
Cell-mediated defect	*Pneumocystis*
	Viruses
	Fungi
	Atypical mycobacteria
	'the rest'

Table 6.2 Organisms commonly associated with different types of impairment of resistance to infection

Bacterial pneumonia

Pneumococcal pneumonia is still the most common community-acquired pneumonic illness in the previously healthy adult. Involvement of one or more lobes in their entirety is characteristic. Splenectomized patients and those suffering from hypogammaglobulinaemia are particularly prone to pneumococcal infection, often of considerable severity. Penicillin G is the antibiotic of choice but the organism is also sensitive to other agents (see Table 6.3).

Mycoplasma pneumoniae and Legionella pneumophila are also seen frequently in the previously healthy, the former usually occurring in patients less than 35 years old, often in localized epidemics, and the latter said to be most common in middle-aged smoking males who are travelling away from home. Infection with *M. pneumoniae* is less likely than pneumococcal pneumonia to be restricted to a single lobe or even only one lung; cold agglutinins are often sought but

Streptococcus pneumoniae	Benzylpenicillin, erythromycin
Haemophilus influenzae	Amoxycillin, co-trimoxazole, cefaclor cefuroxime
Staphylococcus aureus	Flucloxacillin, sodium fusidate
Mycoplasma pneumoniae	Tetracycline, erythromycin
Legionella pneumophila	Erythromycin, rifampicin
Chlamydia psittaci	Tetracycline, co-trimoxazole
Klebsiella pneumoniae	Aminoglycoside and latemoxef disodium, chloramphenicol
Pseudomonas aeruginosa	Aminoglycoside and a ureidopenicillin, ceftazidime
Anaerobic bacteria	Benzylpenicillin and metronidazole
Branhamella catarrhalis	Amoxycillin and clavulanic acid, cefotaxime, cefaclor

Table 6.3   Antibiotic sensitivity of some common pathogens that cause pneumonia

are found in only about 40% of cases, and there is generally only a modest leucocytosis (10 000–12 000 mm^{-3}). A severe systemic illness is common with *Legionella* pneumonia as evidenced by early mental confusion, impaired renal function, gastrointestinal disturbances, hyponatraemia and abnormalities of liver function. Illness caused by this organism is diagnosed more frequently now that it can be isolated in culture; a rapid immunoassay is also available. Both *M. pneumoniae* and *L. pneumophila* are sensitive to erythromycin and tetracycline (Table 6.3).

Infection with *Gram-negative organisms* occurs most commonly in those with some predisposition to infection: for example *Haemophilus influenzae* in the very young or those with hypogammaglobulinaemia; *Klebsiella pneumoniae* in alcoholics; and almost any Gram-negative rod in those who develop a secondary infection while receiving broad-spectrum antibiotic cover for some other condition. *Pseudomonas aeruginosa* is particularly common in patients already requiring mechanical ventilatory support, but it is not always easy to ascertain when it is definitely pathogenic. Infection with more than one organism is common in these circumstances, and antibiotic cover is often chosen with this in mind; a popular combination is an aminoglycoside with a broad-spectrum anti-pseudomonal penicillin (e.g. piperacillin) or, possibly, a cephalosporin (e.g. ceftazidime).

Anaerobic organisms are associated particularly with localized infection and inadequate drainage, e.g. lung abscess, secondary infection of an aspergilloma, or after aspiration of vomit. They are most unlikely to be the cause of a diffuse pneumonia in the absence of other pulmonary pathology. Foul-smelling sputum will be expectorated once drainage has been established, and marked fetor is often present before this, because carious teeth are a common antecedent.

Viral pneumonia

Viral pneumonia, particularly that caused by the influenza group, is more likely than bacterial infection to result in widespread and usually bilateral shadowing. Leucopenia is present in a proportion of cases, and overwhelming pulmonary oedema causing death in a matter of hours occurs occasionally. The chief hazard is secondary infection, usually with *Staphylococcus aureus*, an organism associated particularly with the presence on chest X-ray of multiple thin-walled abscess cavities which may persist as cysts after recovery. The drug treatment of viral pneumonia is disappointing, with the exception of acyclovir for disseminated herpetic infection, usually seen only in the immunocompromised. Antibiotic cover to protect against infection with *S. aureus* should be given, flucloxacillin, sodium fusidate, cefotaxime or lincomycin being worthy of consideration.

Management

Oxygen should be given at a concentration of 35–60% to patients who are cyanosed or distressed. There is negligible risk of depressing respiratory drive, and carbon dioxide retention occurs only in the exhausted and terminally ill. Analgesics are sometimes needed to relieve pleuritic pain and here too there is little risk of drug-induced respiratory depression. Fever, sweating and breathlessness may have resulted in dehydration, so fluids should be encouraged by mouth. Intravenous rehydration may be necessary but over-hydration must be avoided because non-cardiogenic pulmonary oedema (page 54) is a complication of severe pneumonia and can easily be worsened by over-enthusiastic transfusion, especially with normal saline. Oliguria and a low urinary sodium concentration occur with acute hypoxia and incipient circulatory failure as well as with hypovolaemia.

Choice of antibiotic

Many common bacteria causing pneumonia are sensitive to a wide range of antibiotics and so choice of a broad-spectrum drug is often effective, even though the pathogen has not been identified. Organisms with an unusual pattern of sensitivity, antibiotic intolerance by the patient, or the presence of atypical pathogens - particularly in immunocompromised patients - emphasize the importance of securing an accurate microbiological diagnosis if at all possible. In practice, even the most painstaking efforts to identify the organism are unsuccessful in a proportion of patients and, more often, a decision to institute treatment immediately has to be taken on the basis of probability without waiting for the results of culture or immunodiagnostic tests, because the patient is acutely ill or is deteriorating rapidly. Guidelines for the choice of antibiotic in some common clinical situations are given in Tables 6.3 and 6.4.

Patients who fail to respond promptly or who are suffering from an overwhelming infection may require mechanical assistance to ventilation. Here too the decision to intervene is usually taken on clinical grounds - increasing confusion and restlessness (indicative of hypoxia), a rising heart rate, sweating and peripheral vasoconstriction.

Community acquired
A. Previously healthy adult
Streptococcus pneumoniae
Staphylococcus aureus plus virus
Mycoplasma pneumoniae
Legionella pneumophila
Chlamydia psittaci
B. Poor social circumstances, alcohol excess, exposure
Streptococcus pneumoniae
Staphylococcus aureus
Haemophilus influenzae
Klebsiella pneumoniae
Anaerobic bacteria
Hospital acquired
Staphylococcus aureus
Pseudomonas aeruginosa
Escherichia coli
Proteus mirabilis
Branhamella catarrhalis
Anaerobic bacteria

Table 6.4 Common pathogens causing pneumonia in different circumstances

Arterial blood gas tensions measured at this stage are easy to misinterpret because profound hypoxaemia is usually detected and is often greater than the degree of cyanosis would suggest (see page 5). If mechanical ventilation is required, it is wise to assume that the alveolar capillary membrane is damaged and that non-cardiogenic pulmonary oedema is present (see page 54).

Pneumonia in the immunocompromised

Attention has been drawn already to the prevalence of pneumonia in the immunocompromised in general, but it is patients with severe acquired defects of specific immune mechanisms who are most at risk and liable to deteriorate with alarming rapidity. A wide variety of pathogens can be responsible, including not only those discussed already but also organisms usually regarded as non-invasive (e.g. *Branhamella catarrhalis*), or fungi (usually *Candida* in the UK, less commonly *Aspergillus* or *Nocardia*), *Myocobacterium tuberculosis* or atypical mycobacteria, viral infection (particularly cytomegalovirus), and *Pneumocystis carinii*. Interest in the last-named organism has been enhanced by its prevalence in patients with AIDS, when it often occurs with cytomegalovirus infection.

Investigation
The differential diagnosis of fever and pulmonary shadowing in the immunocompromised includes a number of non-infective causes (Table 6.5) and information which may help to clarify the cause is listed in Table 6.6. Infection with more than one organism is common and sometimes one can be isolated but not the other; culture of sputum from the upper airway can confuse the diagnosis because it may contain potential pathogens which differ from the intrapulmonary infection. Invasive investigations such as transtracheal aspiration, fibre-optic bronchoscopy, bronchial lavage, and transbronchial or even open lung biopsy may be necessary, but even then the diagnosis remains obscure in a proportion of patients. The decision to proceed with invasive tests should be taken only *as an emergency* in a centre familiar with such patients and their management. A further argument against over-radical intervention at an early stage is that it probably has little influence on outcome.

Management
The mortality associated with fever and pulmonary

Irradiation

Drug reaction

Graft-versus-host disease

Leucoagglutinin reaction

Tumour

Haemorrhage

Pulmonary oedema

Pulmonary embolism

Undiagnosed after investigation

Table 6.5 Non-infective causes of fever and pulmonary shadowing in the immunocompromised host

Essential history

Nature, time course and current status of antecedent disease

Hospital or community acquired?

Past history of infection/exposure?

Table 6.6 Essential information for the accurate diagnosis of fever and pulmonary shadowing in the immunocompromised host

shadowing in the immunocompromised is high and those who are going to survive are likely to do so if immediate treatment is instituted to combat the common pathogenic bacteria. Empirical treatment for infection with *Pneumocystis carinii* is less defensible because the disease progresses more slowly, antibiotic therapy will be required for a minimum of a fortnight (usually longer), and the incidence of adverse effects is fairly high, particularly in patients with AIDS.

PULMONARY COLLAPSE

Acute massive collapse of the lung occurs abruptly if an inhaled foreign body impacts in a major bronchus. Obstruction by a plug of mucus or blood clot can also occur

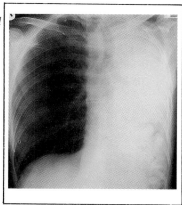

Figure 6.1 Acute massive collapse of the lung. There is gross mediastinal displacement, herniation of the right lung across the mid-line, and elevation of the left hemidiaphragm shown subsequently to be due in part to an incomplete left phrenic paralysis. Unlike the radiological features after pneumonectomy, the ribs are not particularly crowded, there is no bony defect and there is no evidence of extraneous material closing the bronchus.

suddenly, the former particularly common in patients with allergic bronchopulmonary aspergillosis. A bronchus which has been getting gradually narrower as a result of an intra-luminal neoplasm or external compression may finally close completely as a result of mucous impaction, oedema or haemorrhage but the acute event is likely to have been preceded by other symptoms.

Clinical features

Sudden collapse of the lung causes severe dyspnoea, pain, cyanosis, and often impairment of the peripheral circulation. Considerable mediastinal displacement may follow (Figure 6.1), especially in younger subjects, and this contributes to the circulatory disturbances. The symptoms are similar but much less profound if the collapse affects only a lobe, and can be minimal if only the middle lobe or a bronchopulmonary segment is affected. The differential diagnosis includes acute pulmonary embolism, myocardial infarction and spontaneous pneumothorax, but confusion is likely only when the area of collapse is small and the signs are unimpressive. The chest X-ray provides confirmation.

Management

The patient should be sat up and, if tolerated, turned a little so that the affected side is uppermost.

Oxygen, analgesia

Oxygen should be supplied at a concentration of 35–60% and small doses of analgesics given intravenously and titrated against the severity of the pain.

Increasing the humidity

Depending on the cause, percussion and expiratory shaking by an experienced physiotherapist may be sufficient to dislodge the obstruction, but more often this does little more than add to the patient's discomfort and exhaustion. If impaction of mucus is suspected, every effort should be made to increase the humidity of the inspired air (or oxygen). Fifteen to twenty minute periods of inhaling distilled water from an ultrasonic nebulizer may help to liquefy mucous plugs, and treatment can be repeated every couple of hours or so. An alternative which is sometimes effective is the inhalation of hypertonic saline (3 ml nebulized in a stream of compressed air or oxygen), which can be repeated three or four times a day. Patients are unlikely to persevere with this treatment for long because the hypertonic saline irritates mucosal surfaces, particularly the mouth and tongue.

Antibiotics

Pulmonary collapse predisposes to infection, so antibiotics will be needed too unless rapid relief of obstruction and re-expansion of the lung can be achieved by mechanical measures. Antibiotic prophylaxis is controversial because broad-spectrum cover predisposes to infection with organisms which are resistant to treatment, often *Pseudomonas aeruginosa*. Interpreting the results of sputum culture can mislead because organisms isolated from mucus obtained proximal to the obstruction may not be responsible for infection beyond it, and then empirical antibiotic treatment will be needed if there are systemic manifestations such as fever or leucocytosis.

Bronchoscopy

Bronchoscopy should be arranged if a foreign body is

suspected or if the measures outlined above are unsuccessful. General anaesthesia is often preferable to local analgesia because it is easier to proceed to rigid (as distinct from fibre-optic) bronchoscopy if necessary, and many patients will be too distresssed to tolerate the procedure or co-operate while conscious.

Mechanical ventilation

Sometimes it proves impossible to aspirate tenacious mucus, even with the wide-bore suction available through the rigid bronchoscope and in spite of instilling liberal quantities of normal saline. When this occurs, or if the patient is exhausted and distressed by dyspnoea and pain, intubation and mechanical ventilation are necessary. In these cases, humidification should be increased by injecting normal saline down the endotracheal tube (see page 29), which usually results in liquefaction of mucous plugs and re-expansion of the lung.

Patients with lung or lobar collapse of more gradual onset can be treated much more conservatively, management being governed by the nature of the causative lesion.

7.Pulmonary Oedema

Pulmonary oedema exists when extravascular lung water accumulates to excess, either in the alveolar walls or within the alveolar space. The common haemodynamic causes are left ventricular failure secondary to myocardial infarction, systemic hypertension, aortic valve disease, and mitral valve disease. Less common haemodynamic causes include the high pulmonary blood flow of a large left to right shunt (e.g. septal rupture complicating myocardial infarction), a number of congenital cardiac defects, rare tumours of the left atrium causing intermittent obstruction of the mitral valve, and occlusion of pulmonary veins. An elevated pulmonary capillary pressure is common to all these examples, and oedema forms because of this increase in hydrostatic pressure.

Non-cardiogenic pulmonary oedema occurs in the absence of an increase in hydrostatic pressure in the pulmonary capillaries and is attributed to damage affecting both the alveolar epithelium and the capillary endothelium. It develops in association with a wide variety of diverse antecedent conditions (Table 7.1) and its pathogenesis is still uncertain. Unlike the low-protein transudate which accumulates when the hydrostatic pressure is high, non-cardiogenic pulmonary oedema is rich in protein and often progresses to pulmonary fibrosis.

CARDIOGENIC PULMONARY OEDEMA

Clinical features

Dyspnoea and a dry, unproductive cough are the early symptoms, soon followed by worsening dyspnoea, orthopnoea and tachypnoea. The cough becomes

Common	Less common
Major trauma	Pancreatitis
Septicaemia	Pneumonia (often viral)
Fat embolism	Inhaled irritants (including burns)
Aspiration of gastric acid	Blast injury
	Amniotic fluid embolism
	Intravenous narcotic abuse

Table 7.1 Some causes of the adult respiratory distress syndrome

productive and the sputum looser, culminating in the expectoration of pink frothy sputum which represents haemorrhage at alveolar level. Audible wheezing is common and reflects airway narrowing caused by mucosal oedema and congestion; small haemoptyses may occur for the same reason. Signs of cardiac pathology are present in virtually every case, although they may be difficult to elicit if the patient is restless, breathing is noisy and the heart sounds are quiet. The heart is not always enlarged, either on clinical or radiological examination, and abnormalities on the ECG do not necessarily relate to recent pathology. Engorgement of the hilar vessels and prominence of the upper lobe veins are good radiological signs but the latter in particular can be detected only on a film taken with the patient upright. Oedema apparent radiologically is usually symmetrical but is not always so.

Management

Cardiogenic pulmonary oedema will resolve if the pulmonary capillary pressure is lowered, either by reducing the volume of blood entering the lungs or by improving ventricular function. Definitive treatment for the haemodynamic defect will be required but is beyond the scope of this book.

Provided the blood pressure is adequate, the patient should be nursed upright or even sitting in a chair so that gravity aids the relief of pulmonary vascular engorgement.

Oxygen

Oxygen administration helps to relieve dyspnoea and quell anxiety and this too promotes vasodilatation and the transfer of blood out of the pulmonary circulation. Although the arterial carbon dioxide tension is sometimes elevated initially, it is likely to fall rather than rise when hypoxaemia is relieved unless there is severe coincident pulmonary disease.

Diuretics

Diuretics will promote fluid loss unless circulatory or renal failure is extreme. The dose and route of administration depend upon the urgency with which a diuresis is required, the extent of overall fluid retention (is there peripheral oedema too?), and whether an unacceptable reduction in cardiac output can be expected if there is an abrupt reduction in filling pressure. In general, the failing heart changes its performance very little when the pre-load (cardiac filling) is altered, and the output will tend to rise if the after-load (impedance to ejection) is lowered. Conversely, the output of the normal ventricle is markedly influenced by pre-load and to a much lesser extent by after-load. Thus a patient with severe left ventricular damage causing pulmonary oedema and peripheral circulatory failure may only diurese after a large dose of diuretic given intravenously, and the cardiac output is unlikely to fall much if at all as a result of the reduction in intravascular volume. By contrast, a patient with aortic stenosis causing left ventricular failure and pulmonary oedema should be treated much more cautiously, because even a modest reduction in cardiac filling may lower the cardiac output considerably and this in turn impedes perfusion of the hypertrophied myocardium so that catastrophic circulatory failure, heart block or asystole result.

Sedation

Sedation, preferably with an opiate, will relieve anxiety, promote vasodilatation and the relief of pulmonary engorgement, and diminish the tendency of hyperventilation which is probably caused, at least in part, by mechanical stimuli from the engorged pulmonary vascular bed. Sedatives should be avoided if there is severe aortic stenosis because arteriolar dilatation and even a slight reduction in arterial pressure impair the function of the hypertrophied ventricle.

Vasoactive drugs

Vasoactive drugs which reduce pre-load, after-load, or both, or inotropic agents which augment ventricular performance have a role in the management of cardiogenic pulmonary oedema, as do measures for regulating abnormalities of cardiac rhythm.

Mechanical ventilation

Mechanical ventilation should be considered for patients with cardiogenic pulmonary oedema if any aspect of the cardiac pathology is believed to be reversible and if the measures outlined above have proved unsuccessful. It displaces blood from the lungs into the systemic circulation, increases the likelihood of securing a normal arterial oxygen saturation, and removes the work of breathing. The cardiac output is unlikely to fall significantly or may even rise, and a diuresis often follows.

NON-CARDIOGENIC PULMONARY OEDEMA OR ADULT RESPIRATORY DISTRESS SYNDROME (ARDS)

Clinical features

Rapidly worsening dyspnoea is the main symptom but tachypnoea or an inappropriate tachycardia is often manifest before any other abnormality. Arterial hypoxaemia and hypocapnia occur early and the changes are often far more extreme than would be anticipated from symptoms or signs. Physical signs are sparse unless the condition follows direct injury - for example trauma to the chest or inhalation of an irritant, the latter often causing bronchospasm and bronchorrhoea as well as alveolar damage. The chest X-ray usually shows diffuse opacities which rapidly become confluent and are sometimes distributed asymmetrically, depending on cause and recent posture. Considerable functional derangement can exist without much radiological abnormality initially, but changes are usually apparent by the time the diagnosis is suspected.

The syndrome is commonly associated with serious, often rapidly changing pathology affecting other systems and the differential diagnosis of dyspnoea and hypoxaemia includes a wide range of conditions. Pulmonary oedema in the absence of pulmonary venous hypertension is the most important feature but the presence of ARDS is not excluded by coincident cardiac disease, so invasive haemodynamic monitoring or even lung biopsy may be needed to confirm the diagnosis. More often it is assumed on the basis of consistent clinical, radiological and physiological features occurring in the presence of an appropriate antecedent condition.

Management

Treatment is largely empirical and the most important measure is to identify the antecedent condition and to correct it if possible.

Control of infection
The control of infection is of paramount importance and can involve surgical intervention to drain pus as well as the use of antibiotics. Infection developing in a patient already suffering from ARDS should be identified and treated very vigorously because the already high mortality is roughly doubled by its presence. Prophylactic antibiotics are sometimes recommended but this is likely to result in the appearance of resistant organisms.

Corticosteroids
There is some evidence that corticosteroids given early and in large doses have a beneficial effect on the evolution of

ARDS, but this policy does not have universal support. The recommended regimen is methylprednisolone $30\,mg\,kg^{-1}$ given by slow intravenous injection and repeated once or twice in the first 48 hours. Corticosteroid treatment should not be prolonged beyond this time because there is no evidence to suggest that it promotes resolution of oedema or impedes fibrosis, but there is an increased risk of complications such as infection or gastrointestinal ulceration.

Oxygen

Supportive treatment consists of measures to improve oxygenation, to maintain the cardiac output and to keep the pulmonary capillary pressure as low as possible. Oxygen is given initially at concentrations of up to 60% (the highest available with most simple masks), but mechanical ventilation is needed in a high proportion of cases. Oxygen toxicity has been implicated in the pathogenesis of ARDS, and the use of positive end-expiratory pressure (PEEP) or spontaneous ventilation with continuous positive airway pressure (CPAP) may mean that a lower inspired oxygen concentration is adequate. Measures such as these are best carried out in an intensive care unit with appropriate monitoring.

8.Haemoptysis, Pulmonary Haemorrhage and Pulmonary Embolism

HAEMOPTYSIS

Haemoptysis, the expectoration of blood or blood-stained sputum, varies in severity from the trifling blood loss associated with acute infection to massive, life-threatening haemorrhage caused by the erosion of a major vessel, e.g. by neoplasm, or deep-seated destructive pulmonary infection such as bronchiectasis, cavitating pulmonary tuberculosis or an infected aspergilloma. Investigation and treatment vary, depending on cause and severity, and only severe haemorrhage will be considered here.

Clinical features

Haemorrhage is sometimes preceded by audible bubbling and the patient notices a salt taste as soon as blood enters the mouth. There may be little or no coughing if there is rapid bleeding, because the blood merely wells up through the larynx. Characteristically it is bright-red and frothy, and haemorrhage of this magnitude can usually be distinguished without difficulty from haematemesis or bleeding from the upper respiratory tract. The magnitude of associated respiratory distress depends upon the degree of underlying pulmonary damage and the extent to which blood contaminates the remaining lung or obstructs the major airways. Blood loss can be sufficient to precipitate circulatory failure, but tachycardia and vasoconstriction may be no more than a manifestation of the fear which is inevitable with haemoptysis of this magnitude.

Management

Urgent admission to hospital should be arranged and the

patient should travel with the affected side dependent, if this can be identified. The semi-prone position promotes drainage of blood which does reach the trachea or pharynx and so minimizes contamination of the rest of the lung, but the conscious breathless patient prefers to sit up.

Oxygen
Oxygen should be given in high concentration and it may be reasonable to accept the calculated risk of a small dose of an opiate given intravenously to minimize restlessness and lessen any urgent desire to cough unproductively.

Initial investigations
On admission, blood should be cross-matched and a transfusion given if necessary. An immediate chest X-ray sometimes provides almost incontrovertible evidence of the source of bleeding but this is not so in the presence of generalized disease such as bronchiectasis or tuberculosis (Figure 8.1) or if there has been such extensive aspiration of blood that there is radiological shadowing on both sides. Many patients will volunteer an opinion on which side the blood originates from, and their impression is usually correct.

Bronchoscopy
If the diagnosis is in doubt, immediate fibre-optic bronchoscopy will usually identify the source of bleeding,

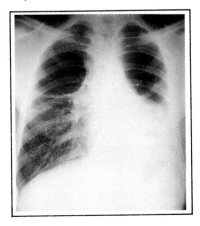

Figure 8.1 Bilateral apical cavities and extensive left lower zone consolidation in a patient who presented with haemoptysis.

although the view can be obscured by active haemorrhage or, if bleeding has ceased, all the segmental orifices appear equally contaminated with blood-stained mucus.

If massive bleeding continues or recurs, rigid bronchoscopy under general anaesthesia should be considered. Measures which can be implemented then include the application of pressure to a proximal bleeding source, lavage with ice-cold saline, or the insertion of a bronchus blocker to isolate the source of haemorrhage. A further alternative is insertion of a double-lumen endobronchial tube so that a clear airway can be preserved on one side while the other lumen permits aspiration of blood as necessary.

Invasive management

Invasive measures for the control of pulmonary haemorrhage include ligation of the bronchial vessels at thoracotomy or their embolization under radiological control.

PULMONARY HAEMORRHAGE

Haemorrhage into the alveolar walls and spaces presents a totally different picture, occurring either in isolation (idiopathic pulmonary haemosiderosis) or in association with renal damage, when there are circulating antibodies to glomerular basement membrane and the deposition of immune complexes in both the lungs and the kidneys (Goodpasture's syndrome).

Clinical features

Breathlessness of fairly sudden onset is characteristic, usually developing over a matter of hours and not associated with either pain or fever, and only with haemoptysis in the most severe cases. Tachycardia, tachypnoea and cyanosis result, and there is widespread radiological opacification which may be discrete or confluent (Figure 8.2). Patients who present urgently are likely to have widespread confluent pulmonary shadowing

Figure 8.2 Diffuse pulmonary haemorrhage.

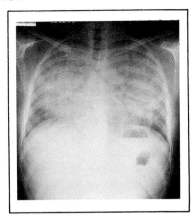

but, unlike other causes of profound hypoxaemia with such extensive radiological change, the degree of respiratory distress is less than might be anticipated, possibly because there is no increase in metabolic demand and little derangement of pulmonary haemodynamics.

Investigations which suggest or support the diagnosis include progressive fall in the haemoglobin concentration in the absence of alternative sources of blood loss or evidence of haemolysis, and associated renal dysfunction, again without other cause. The presence of iron-laden macrophages in sputum or in specimens obtained by bronchial lavage is diagnostic. Measurement of the transfer factor (diffusing capacity of the lungs for carbon monoxide) is helpful when there has been recent bleeding, because the presence of haemoglobin in large amounts in the alveoli increases the uptake of carbon monoxide with the result that the measured value is very high. This elevation of the transfer factor can be obscured by coincident reduction in the size of the alveolar space to which the test gas gains access, but lung volume can be measured easily at the same time by helium dilution, and then the transfer coefficient (Kco) can be calculated too. The transfer coefficient, derived by dividing the transfer factor by alveolar volume, is also elevated after recent pulmonary haemorrhage.

Management

The treatment of idiopathic pulmonary haemosiderosis is solely supportive, there being little or no evidence of benefit with either corticosteroids or immunosuppresive regimens. Goodpasture's syndrome can however be treated, often with excellent results, by plasmapheresis, followed, if necessary, by immunotherapy. Treatment becomes a matter of urgency if either renal or pulmonary function is deteriorating very rapidly.

Those with profound pulmonary haemorrhage will require mechanical ventilation and probably blood transfusion too. In the most severe cases the haemorrhage is so profuse that blood enters the airway, causing both obstruction and impaired gas exchange.

PULMONARY EMBOLISM

The consequences of pulmonary embolism vary in severity from a small peripheral infarct, which may pass unnoticed, to major obstruction of the proximal pulmonary arteries resulting in cardiovascular collapse and sudden death. The differential diagnosis of peripheral pulmonary emboli causing infarction is from collapse or consolidation, whereas central obstruction to pulmonary circulation (acute massive pulmonary embolism) is confused most readily with myocardial infarction.

Clinical features

Prolonged immobility, recent surgery or delivery, pulmonary congestion, and states of hypercoagulability of the blood are the common factors predisposing to pulmonary embolism. Antecedent deep venous thrombosis is usually present but often with no focal signs and manifest only, if at all, by slight fever and tachycardia. These warning signs are useful but present in only a proportion of patients who subsequently suffer an embolus. Chest pain, slight breathlessness and small haemoptyses are the traditional

Figure 8.3 (a) Chest X-ray after acute massive pulmonary embolism; there is marked avascularity of the right lower zone. (b) Pulmonary angiogram of the same patient.

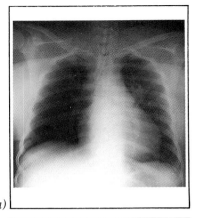

(a)

(b)

features of a small peripheral pulmonary embolus causing infarction. Extreme dyspnoea, faintness and circulatory collapse occur with acute massive pulmonary embolism, and conscious patients may notice chest pain indistinguishable from angina pectoris (and, indeed, probably caused by acute myocardial ischaemia). Chest X-ray (Figure 8.3) and ECG (Figure 8.4) help to distinguish pulmonary embolism from other causes of chest pain or collapse but venography, ventilation/perfusion scanning or pulmonary angiography are likely to be needed for confirmation.

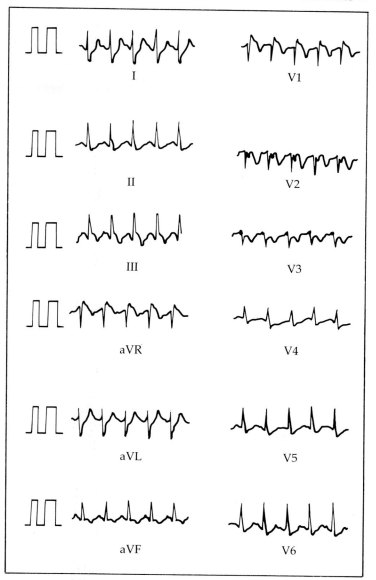

Figure 8.4 ECG recorded from a 17-year-old female after acute massive pulmonary embolism.

Management

Small peripheral pulmonary emboli are treated with intravenous heparin, initially a bolus injection of 5000 units, followed by a continuous infusion of 40 000 units per day using a syringe pump. Adequacy of anticoagulation is monitored using the kaolin cephalin clotting time. Recurrence may be prevented by the use of oral anticoagulants.

Massive pulmonary embolism is confirmed by pulmonary angiography and treated by infusion of either streptokinase or urokinase via the catheter or embolectomy.

9.Pneumothorax, Lung Cysts and Bronchopleural Fistula

PNEUMOTHORAX

Pneumothorax, haemopneumothorax and pulmonary contusion are common after chest trauma and are often associated with other injuries which influence management. This chapter deals only with pneumothoraces occurring spontaneously.

Clinical features

Chest pain of sudden onset followed rapidly by shortness of breath is the classic description, but pain can be absent or minimal when a pneumothorax complicates pre-existing pulmonary disease, and the degree of breathlessness is determined by how far the lung collapses and whether lung function is already compromised. The physical signs of a large pneumothorax are easy to elicit but a pneumothorax is more difficult to detect if:

1. The chest is hyperinflated and the breath sounds faint, as in emphysema or very severe asthma;

2. There is already asymmetrical lung pathology;

3. The pneumothorax is small or loculated, e.g. beneath the lung.

The chest X-ray is usually diagnostic but a shallow pneumothorax can be missed unless a film is taken in full expiration, when the lung edge is forced away from the chest wall. A pneumothorax under considerable tension must sometimes be drained before an X-ray can be obtained because the combination of pulmonary collapse and distortion of the mediastinum are causing life-threatening circulatory failure. If there is any possibility that the air is loculated as well as under tension (Figure 9.1), its location is best determined by the combination of visible over-distension of the chest and hyper-resonance to percussion. Even these physical signs will be inapparent if there is surgical emphysema too, and then a fine diagnostic needle in both sides of the chest must be used if there really is no time to await radiological examination.

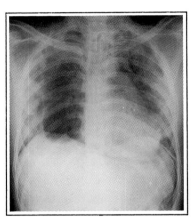

Figure 9.1 Loculated tension pneumothoraces and surgical emphysema in a patient with ARDS requiring mechanical ventilation.

Management

Questions to be considered before deciding that a pneumothorax requires drainage include:

1. How large is it?

2. How long has it been present?

3. Is respiration embarrassed at rest? On exertion?

4. Is the lung either tethered or unable to collapse because of emphysema, extensive fibrosis or consolidation so that the air collects in pockets?

5. If loculated, will placement of a drain be easy?

6. Will any other aspect of patient management (e.g. requirement for mechanical ventilation) influence the need for pleural drainage?

Shallow pneumothorax (less than 20%)
This will absorb in 3–6 weeks without treatment, provided the site from which the air escaped has sealed. However, even in the otherwise healthy, it is rare to adopt an entirely non-interventionist policy. Air can be evacuated from the pleural space by aspiration or by establishing an under-water seal drain. The former is less invasive and allows early mobilization but there is a risk of late recurrence of the pneumothorax. Insertion of a drain is more painful, immobilizes the patient and carries a higher risk of causing vascular or pulmonary damage.

If aspiration is chosen, it should be carried out with a fine-bore catheter to avoid damaging the lung surface. Removal of 0.5 to 1 litre of air should suffice to eliminate all but a trace of a pneumothorax which initially occupies 20% of the cavity, and there is no need to measure intrapleural pressure routinely. A further X-ray should be taken after a few hours to confirm that the air is not re-accumulating. If it is, or if there is a subsequent recurrence on the same side, pleural drainage is probably preferable to further aspiration because the presence of the tube encourages the formation of adhesions. The steps for establishing an under-water seal drain are described on page 69 and illustrated in Figure 9.3. Patients who present with recurrent or bilateral pneumothoraces should be considered for pleural surgery.

Deep pneumothorax (more than 20%)
A deep pneumothorax is more likely to be associated with dyspnoea, and conventional management is to insert a chest drain. However, a case can be made for aspiration to convert the deep pneumothorax into a shallow space and then allowing the remainder of the air to reabsorb spontaneously.

Figure 9.2 Re-expansion pulmonary oedema following drainage of a large pneumothorax which had been present for about a week. (a) On admission. (b) 12 hours later.

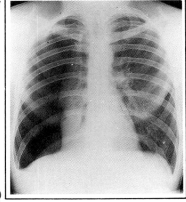

(a)

(b)

Unilateral pulmonary oedema is a rare but dangerous complication after drainage of a large pneumothorax which has been present for more than 48 hours (Figure 9.2). It is heralded by vigorous coughing as the chest drain is inserted, followed by rapid cardiovascular collapse. The cause of collapse is fluid loss into the lung tissue, and careful transfusion, monitored by measurement of the central venous pressure, is the appropriate treatment. A diuretic is *not* indicated and atropine is ineffective. Although the risk of this catastrophe is slight, a case can be made for not draining a large pneumothorax which has been present for some days if the patient is not distressed at rest. Alternatively, the chest can be aspirated to remove some of the air initially and then either further aspiration, or insertion of a drain, can be considered later.

Tension pneumothorax

This requires immediate intercostal drainage and it may be necessary as a matter of urgency to insert a wide-bore intravenous cannula into the chest while preparations for the more invasive procedure are completed. This preliminary cannulation may be just sufficient to lessen the cardiovascular consequences of the tension pneumothorax but will be insufficient to allow much air to escape, and sustained improvement will only follow insertion of a drain of adequate size attached to an under-water seal.

Although there has in the past been enthusiasm for draining the pleural cavity through the second interspace anteriorly, this approach is uncomfortable, relatively inefficient and leaves an unsightly scar. There is a general preference now for a lateral approach from the lower intercostal spaces, a little anterior to the mid-axillary line (Figure 9.3a). The important prerequisites for successful placement of a pleural drain are:

1. Support the patient in a comforable, upright posture.

2. Cleanse the operating site. Infiltrate with local anaesthetic to the pleura and check that the needle passes through to the pleural cavity by aspirating air. Wait until the local anaesthetic takes effect.

3. Make a 2 cm incision in the skin following the upper edge of the rib (Figure 9.3b). Open the layer of tissues down to the pleura with a pair of blunt dissecting forceps (Figure 9.3c).

4. Insert the trochar and cannula obliquely through the prepared site, pointing towards the apex of the lung and using only slight pressure to pierce the pleura, with the trochar guard or forceps clipped onto the cannula to prevent it being pushed too far into the chest (Figure 9.3d).

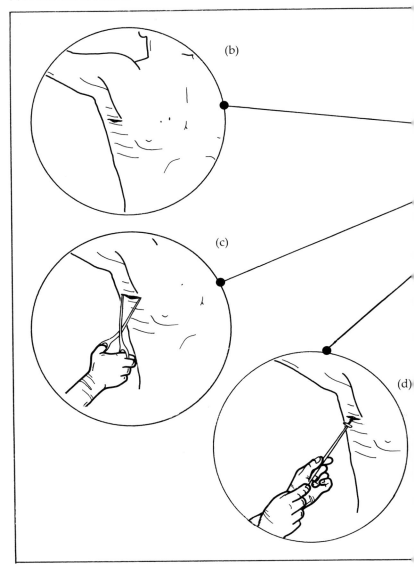

Figure 9.3 Steps in the insertion of an intercostal drain. (a) Selection of site. A = Fifth intercostal space in the mid-axillary line. B = Second intercostal space in the mid-clavicular line. (b) Making the incision.

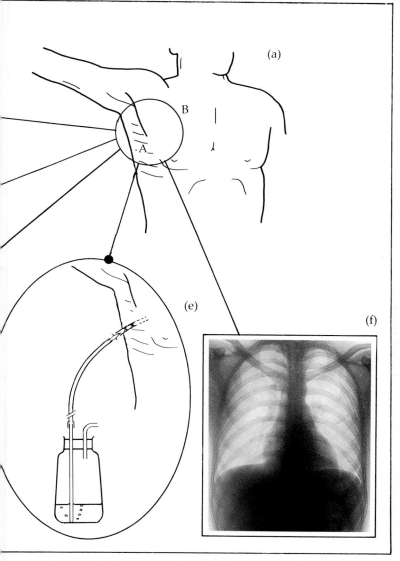

(c) Opening the tissues to the pleura. (d) Insertion of trochar and cannula. (e) Drainage of pneumothorax via an under-water seal. (f) Confirmation by X-ray.

5. Advance the catheter off the trochar towards the apex of the lung and attach it to an under-water seal (Figure 9.3e). Stitch a black silk purse-string suture around the incision and tie it around the catheter to hold it in place. Apply a small amount of strapping to cover the site of insertion. Check that all connections are air-tight and that the drainage system is bubbling during coughing or expiration.

6. Take a chest X-ray to ensure that the drain is in good position, ideally at the apex of the lung in most cases (Figure 9.3f).

Once the drain has been correctly sited and connected to an underwater seal (or to a non-return valve), air should escape freely and the lung will start to re-expand. If air stops escaping and yet the lung remains deflated, it is worth asking the patient to try to take a few deep breaths or even cough. Pain limits co-operation with this manoeuvre but it is often sufficient to overcome the initial resistance of the lung to re-expansion and further progress will then be rapid.

If the lung fails to expand and there is a brisk air leak, suction can be applied to the drain (-20 to -50 cm of water) or, in exceptional circumstances, a second drain may be needed.

Loculated pneumothorax

This is much more difficult to treat safely and successfully and, unless it is causing serious interference with respiration, is often best left alone. If urgent drainage is necessary, consider inserting an intravenous catheter through the chest wall at the point of maximum distension and resonance. A lateral chest film as well as a P-A or A-P view may help to locate the air pocket. If it is clearly difficult to enter, use of an intravenous catheter will minimize the extent of damage caused if the lung is punctured or if other viscera are perforated. If the catheter has to be inserted with the patient lying supine, remember that the diaphragm (and therefore the abdominal contents) are much higher than in the upright subject.

LUNG CYSTS

A large lung cyst can mimic a loculated pneumothorax but usually the distinction can be made by observing the rounded shape of the medial edge on the chest film. The cyst will deflate unless it is in communication with the air passages and it will only enlarge rapidly if:

1. The communication acts as a one-way valve.

2. Positive pressure is applied to the lungs (or the patient is decompressed).

3. The inert gas within the cyst (nitrogen) is replaced by a more soluble agent (e.g. nitrous oxide) which enters the cyst more rapidly than the nitrogen can escape.

Large lung cysts compress and distort the surrounding lung and occasionally present as a respiratory or cardiovascular crisis. The only effective immediate treatment is to insert a drain into the cyst, accepting that this automatically creates a fistula. Undesirable though this may be, the consequences are of negligible hazard as long as the air can escape freely. It is highly unlikely that the communication between the cyst and airway is so large that more than a small proportion of tidal air will escape preferentially through the fistula, because otherwise the cyst would not have enlarged and become tense in the first place. Once respiratory distress has been relieved and cardiovascular stability has returned, the patient should be referred for a thoracic surgical opinion.

Herniated viscera, especially the stomach, can be mistaken for an encysted tension pneumothorax or lung cyst. Here attempts at 'pleural drainage' can have disastrous consequences. Features which should arouse suspicion include a history of blunt chest or abdominal trauma, even many years previously, abdominal symptoms such as pain or vomiting, hypotension and tachycardia out of proportion to the apparent magnitude of the 'pneumothorax', and atypical radiological appearances (Figure 9.4). If the diagnosis is considered, an attempt can be made to pass a nasogastric tube and subsequently locate its tip radiologically, or observe the distribution of a bolus of contrast medium. This may prove impossible because of distortion; then fine-needle aspiration of the cavity can be considered, which may locate fluid of acid pH, so confirming that urgent thoracotomy must be arranged.

BRONCHOPLEURAL FISTULA

This term refers correctly to a communication between the pleural cavity and the bronchial tree, but is often used loosely to describe any communication between the pleural cavity and the lung, even at alveolar level. The implications of the two conditions are so different that the term is better used in the specific rather than the general sense.

Air leaking from the surface of the lung at alveolar level will accumulate in the pleural space, ultimately causing pulmonary collapse and mediastinal displacement. Once drained, the tension in the pleural space disappears and the volume of air leaving the chest by this route is usually small by comparison with tidal ventilation. Even if the patient requires mechanical ventilation, it is exceptional for air to escape from the peripheral parts of the lung in such volume that adequate alveolar ventilation cannot be maintained. Air loss through the chest wall will be augmented if suction is applied to the drain and, if there is any doubt about the adequacy of alveolar ventilation, suction should be avoided if possible, particularly during mechanical ventilation.

If a major bronchus communicates with the pleural space, catastrophic respiratory insufficiency will result very quickly - partly because tension builds up very rapidly in the

Figure 9.4 Congenital diaphragmatic hernia with the stomach occupying much of the left hemithorax.

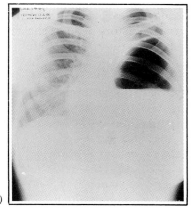

(a)

(b)

pleural space (and air usually also escapes into the tissues causing surgical emphysema too) and partly because the orifice of the distal bronchus is often obstructed by distortion, mucus, blood, etc. As a result, alveolar ventilation is bound to be inadequate and any attempt at positive pressure ventilation will merely enhance the egress of air through the fistula. Immediate management consists of insertion of a large-bore chest drain and isolation of the fistula by endobronchial intubation, usually followed by urgent thoracotomy. These two extremes - air leaking into the pleural space from the surface of the lung, and disruption of a major bronchus - represent the ends of a spectrum.

Management of the individual case depends on an assessment of:

1. The size of the air leak.

2. Its location within the bronchopulmonary tree.

3. Whether the remaining lung tissue is healthy.

Figure 9.5 Bronchopleural fistula after pneumonectomy. (a) Air-fluid level and some contralateral shadowing. (b) Markedly increased contralateral shadowing associated with a fall in the fluid level.

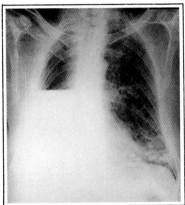

(a)

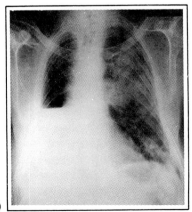

(b)

Post-pneumonectomy

The development of a bronchopleural fistula after pneumonectomy is a special case, in that the pneumonectomy space fills with fluid postoperatively and disruption of the stump allows this to enter the airway and soil the remaining lung (Figure 9.5). A major dehiscence causes sudden dyspnoea accompanied by coughing and the expectoration of, characteristically, thin brown fluid; the associated hypoxia rapidly causes circulatory collapse. Posture to minimize further entry of fluid into the airway and external drainage of the pneumonectomy space are the immediate requirements.

10. Chest Wall and Respiratory Muscle Defects

A miscellaneous group of conditions interfere with
respiration because of weakness, deformity or immobility of
the chest wall (Tables 10.1 and 10.2).

High spinal cord injury

Poliomyelitis

Acute infectious polyneuritis

Myasthenia gravis

Organo-phosphorus insecticide poisoning

Hereditary or acquired myopathy

Table 10.1   Some neuromuscular causes of respiratory insufficiency

Chest wall trauma

Kyphoscoliosis

Pott's disease of the spine (with deformity)

Ankylosing spondylitis

Congenital rib cage anomalies

Table 10.2   Some skeletal causes of respiratory insufficiency

Chest trauma is the most common antecedent of
respiratory insufficiency associated with a skeletal defect,
with or without additional lung injury. The extent of rib
fractures can be difficult to assess radiologically unless
special views are taken, and paradoxical movement is
apparent only if ribs are broken in more than one place so
leaving a flail segment, or if the underlying lung is difficult to
inflate (collapse, consolidation or partial bronchial

occlusion). Major trauma of this type is often associated with other injuries but a minority of patients have only isolated chest wall injury, possibly superimposed on pre-existing pulmonary disease, and management is concerned primarily with sustaining adequate ventilation. Conditions which should be suspected if apparently limited chest trauma is accompanied or followed by inappropriately severe respiratory distress are listed in Table 10.3.

Fat embolism

Adult respiratory distress syndrome

Ruptured bronchus

Ruptured diaphragm

Table 10.3   Causes of disproportionate dyspnoea after chest wall trauma

RESPIRATORY MUSCLE WEAKNESS

Clinical features

The severity of symptoms depends in part on the rapidity with which the weakness has developed. Long-standing weakness, for example after poliomyelitis, can cause a profound reduction in vital capacity but only modest impairment of exercise tolerance. A trifling respiratory illness or even an inappropriate dose of sedation can be life-threatening in such patients and they require far more careful observation than their symptoms or the magnitude of any intercurrent illness would normally warrant.

Similar care is required in the presence of an acutely paralysing illness such as myasthenia gravis, infectious polyneuritis or poisoning with cholinesterase inhibitors (organo-phosphorus insecticides). Profound weakness of the limbs, trunk and facial muscles is often far more apparent than respiratory symptoms to both patient and observer, and 'unexpected' respiratory arrest occurs as a result. Conversely, however, respiratory insufficiency is occasionally the presenting or dominant feature of multiple sclerosis or motor neurone disease. Regular measurement of the vital capacity will alert the observer to the magnitude of the respiratory weakness if the symptoms are unobtrusive, values less than $10 \, \text{ml kg}^{-1}$ in the previously healthy indicating that respiratory insufficiency is probable and that coughing will be ineffective. Far lower values can be tolerated by those with chronic weakness, but, here too, serial measurement or a comparison of vital capacity with values recorded previously will usually indicate when respiratory failure is imminent. A marked accentuation in symptoms and a simultaneous reduction in vital capacity when moving from the upright to the supine position are characteristic of diaphragmatic weakness. Such patients should be nursed upright if at all possible.

Management

Specific treatment, e.g. for myasthenia gravis, cholinergic crisis or poisoning by cholinesterase inhibitors, may be appropriate, but, if respiratory disease is apparent or the vital capacity is less than $7 \, \text{ml kg}^{-1}$, intubation and mechanical ventilation should be considered as well. Mechanical ventilation should be instituted early for acute, progressive disease such as polyneuritis or poliomyelitis because there is a risk of associated bulbar weakness and hence aspiration of saliva or food into the lungs. Excessive salivation is a feature of several of the acutely paralysing illnesses and this too adds to the risk of aspiration. Early tracheostomy is indicated if the weakness is expected to persist for days or weeks, but the long-term prognosis should be considered carefully before embarking on mechanical support for patients with chronic and largely irreversible disease such as progressive myopathy, multiple sclerosis or motor neurone disease.

CHEST WALL DEFORMITY

Clinical features

Here, too, symptoms are often few until disability is

extreme and it is not unusual for patients to present for the first time in respiratory or even cardiac failure. Scoliosis of early onset (below 5 years of age), congenital defects of the ribs, and associated muscle weakness carry a particularly adverse prognosis. Pulmonary as well as extrapulmonary disease is present in some patients: pulmonary fibrosis secondary to previous tuberculosis or ankylosing spondylitis, airways obstruction complicating the pulmonary hypertension of severe scoliosis, or inadequate growth and development of the lung in those with congenital defects. Transitory, reversible airways obstruction in patients with a severe extrapulmonary restrictive defect also occurs, either as a manifestation of bronchial engorgement secondary to heart failure or in response to an acute respiratory infection, when the obstruction is more apparent than usual because of the small size of the air passages.

Management

Carbon dioxide retention is likely to accompany hypoxaemia and so oxygen should be given only in controlled concentrations, monitored by serial estimations of arterial blood gas tensions. Diuretics are usually required and bronchodilator drugs are helpful sometimes, but corticosteroids are only occasionally of value and can cause deterioration because of fluid retention. This is one of the few circumstances in which a bronchodilator administered with intermittent positive pressure breathing is likely to be more effective than use of a nebulized solution with unassisted ventilation. These conventional measures often achieve only mediocre improvement, probably because mechanical inefficiency, respiratory muscle fatigue and nocturnal hypoventilation are of greater importance in perpetuating respiratory insufficiency than minor degrees of airflow limitation.

Non-invasive mechanical ventilation (e.g. negative pressure ventilation with a tank ventilator), followed by long-term nocturnal ventilatory support on a domiciliary basis, gives good results in these patients even when cardiac and respiratory failure appear intransigent in the face of conventional measures. If these facilities are not available and respiratory insufficiency is life threatening, intubation and mechanical ventilation should be instituted initially. Tracheostomy should be avoided if at all possible because it interferes with the less invasive negative-pressure techniques, and its subsequent closure may prove difficult because of the very limited ventilatory reserves. If extubation and adequate spontaneous ventilation cannot be achieved, negative pressure ventilation should be considered and arrangements made for transfer to an appropriate centre if necessary.

Further Reading

1. Brewis RAL.
    Lecture Notes on Respiratory Disease. Oxford: Blackwell
    Scientific, 1980.

2. Crofton JW, Douglas AC.
    Respiratory Diseases, 3rd edn. Oxford : Blackwell Scientific,
    1981.

3. Emerson P, ed.
    Thoracic Medicine. Guildford : Butterworths, 1981.

4. Weatherall DJ, Leadingham JGG, Warrell DA.
    Oxford Textbook of Medicine. London : Oxford University Press,
    1983.

Index

Page numbers in *italics* refer to Figures Letter *t* after page numbers refers to Tables